MAIN SANCHEZ

Transform Your Body in 30 Days

The Ultimate Fitness Challenge

Contents

1

INTRODUCTION

30-Day Fitness Challenge:

Welcome to "Transform Your Body in 30 Days: The Ultimate Fitness Challenge". This book is designed to help you achieve your fitness goals in just 30 days. A 30-day fitness challenge is a compact and intense program designed to provide fast and visible results. It's a perfect way to jump-start your fitness journey or to push yourself to the next level.

The 30-day fitness challenge is designed to work because it sets achievable goals in a short period of time, allowing you to see progress quickly and maintain momentum. This, in turn, provides you with the motivation and confidence to continue your fitness journey long after the challenge is over.

The benefits of completing a 30-day fitness challenge are

numerous. Not only will you see physical changes in your body, such as improved muscle tone, increased strength and endurance, and decreased body fat, but you'll also experience an improved sense of mental and emotional well-being. A regular fitness routine can help reduce stress, improve mood, and increase self-confidence.

Before you begin your 30-day fitness challenge, it's important to set realistic goals. Think about what you want to achieve in the next 30 days, whether it's losing weight, building muscle, or simply becoming more active. It's also important to remember that everyone's fitness journey is different, and it's okay to start small and work your way up.

Preparing mentally and physically for the challenge is key to its success. This means taking the time to plan your workouts, prepare healthy meals, and set aside time each day for exercise. It's also important to focus on developing a positive mindset and to be kind to yourself as you work towards your goals. Remember, this challenge is about progress, not perfection, and every step forward is a step in the right direction.

What is a 30-day fitness challenge and why it works:

A 30-day fitness challenge is a comprehensive fitness program that is completed in a 30-day time frame. The program usually involves a combination of exercise and nutrition, and is designed to provide fast and visible results. The 30-day time frame provides a sense of urgency and helps to maintain motivation and focus, as well as providing a sense of accomplishment once the challenge is completed.

The 30-day fitness challenge works because it sets achievable goals within a short period of time. This allows individuals to see progress quickly and maintain momentum, which helps to keep them motivated and focused on their goals. Additionally, the structured nature of the challenge provides accountability, as individuals have to commit to the program for a set period of time.

The challenge also works because it forces individuals to make healthy choices and prioritize their fitness. For many people, finding the time and motivation to exercise and eat healthily can be a challenge. However, the structure and accountability of a 30-day fitness challenge makes it easier to make these healthy choices, and to stick to them for the duration of the challenge.

In addition to the physical benefits of exercise, such as improved muscle tone, increased strength and endurance, and decreased body fat, the 30-day fitness challenge also provides numerous mental and emotional benefits. Regular exercise has been shown to reduce stress, improve mood, and increase self-confidence, and the structure and focus of a fitness challenge can help to amplify these benefits.

In conclusion, the 30-day fitness challenge works because it provides a structured and comprehensive program that allows individuals to see progress quickly, maintain motivation and focus, and make healthy choices that can have a lasting impact on their health and wellness.

The benefits of completing a 30-day fitness challenge:

Physical Improvements: A 30-day fitness challenge can provide fast and visible physical improvements, such as increased muscle tone, improved strength and endurance, and decreased body fat. This can lead to improved overall health and wellness, and can help to boost self-confidence and self-esteem.

Mental and Emotional Well-being: Regular exercise has been shown to reduce stress and improve mood, and a structured fitness challenge can amplify these benefits. Completing a fitness challenge can also increase self-confidence and provide a sense of accomplishment and satisfaction.

Better Habits: A 30-day fitness challenge can help individuals to develop healthier habits, such as regular exercise and a balanced diet. These habits can have a lasting impact on overall health and wellness, and can help to prevent chronic health conditions, such as heart disease, type 2 diabetes, and certain types of cancer.

Increased Motivation: Completing a fitness challenge can increase motivation and provide a sense of achievement, which can inspire individuals to continue their fitness journey. The structure and accountability of the challenge can also help to maintain focus and motivation, even after the challenge is completed.

Improved Mindset: A positive and focused mindset is key to success in any fitness challenge. Completing a 30-day fitness challenge can help to develop a growth mindset, which is characterized by a belief in personal growth and the ability to overcome challenges. This mindset can be applied to all areas of life, leading to improved overall well-being and success.

Better Sleep: Regular exercise has been shown to improve sleep quality and help individuals to fall asleep more easily. The benefits of better sleep can have a positive impact on overall health and well-being, including improved mood, increased energy, and better cognitive function.

Increased Energy: Exercise is known to increase energy levels, and completing a 30-day fitness challenge can help to amplify these effects. The increased energy levels can help to improve overall health and well-being, and can make it easier to tackle daily challenges with greater ease and effectiveness.

In conclusion, the benefits of completing a 30-day fitness challenge are numerous and can have a lasting impact on overall health and well-being. Whether you're looking to improve physical fitness, mental and emotional well-being, or simply to develop healthier habits, a 30-day fitness challenge is a great place to start.

Setting realistic goals for the 30-day fitness challenge:

Identify your goals: The first step in setting realistic goals for your 30-day fitness challenge is to identify what you want to achieve. This could be anything from losing weight, building muscle, or simply becoming more active. Write down your goals and keep them in mind as you plan your challenge.

Make SMART goals: Once you have identified your goals, it's important to make them SMART - Specific, Measurable, Achievable, Relevant, and Time-bound. This will help to ensure that your goals are realistic and attainable within the 30-day time frame. For example, instead of setting a goal to "lose weight," set a goal to "lose 5 pounds in 30 days."

Be realistic: While it's important to set challenging goals, it's also important to be realistic. Setting goals that are too ambitious can lead to frustration and disappointment, and may result in you giving up before the challenge is complete. Consider your current fitness level and work within your capabilities.

Consider your lifestyle: Your goals should be achievable within the context of your current lifestyle. For example, if you have a demanding work schedule and family commitments, it may not be realistic to set a goal to exercise for two hours every day. Consider what you can realistically fit into your schedule, and set your goals accordingly.

Consider your resources: Consider the resources you have available to you as you set your goals. For example, if you don't have access to a gym, you may need to set goals that can be achieved using bodyweight exercises or with minimal equipment.

Be flexible: Finally, it's important to be flexible and adapt your goals if necessary. If you encounter any roadblocks or challenges during the 30-day challenge, it's important to be able to adjust your goals as needed to ensure that you stay on track.

In conclusion, setting realistic goals for your 30-day fitness challenge is key to success. By making SMART goals, considering your lifestyle and resources, and being flexible, you can ensure that your goals are achievable and that you can successfully complete the challenge.

Preparing mentally and physically for the 30-day fitness challenge:

Build a support system: Surrounding yourself with supportive family and friends can help to provide encouragement and motivation during the challenge. Consider reaching out to friends or joining a fitness community to connect with others who are also taking on the challenge.

Get organized: Make sure that you have everything you need to complete the challenge, including workout clothes, equipment, and healthy food options. Create a plan that fits into your schedule, and make sure that you allocate enough time for exercise, rest, and recovery.

Gradually increase physical activity: If you're new to exercise, or if you haven't been physically active for some time, it's important to gradually increase physical activity to avoid injury. Start with gentle workouts and gradually increase the intensity and duration of your sessions as your body adapts.

Focus on nutrition: A healthy diet is essential for success in any fitness challenge. Focus on eating a balanced diet that includes plenty of fruits and vegetables, lean proteins, and whole grains. Consider tracking your food intake to ensure that you're consuming the right amount of calories and nutrients to support your goals.

Practice mindfulness and relaxation techniques: Exercise can be stressful, especially if you're pushing yourself to reach new goals. Incorporating mindfulness and relaxation techniques into your routine can help to reduce stress and improve overall well-being. This can include practices like meditation, deep breathing, and yoga.

Get enough sleep: Sleep is essential for recovery and rejuvenation, and is particularly important during a fitness challenge. Make sure to get enough sleep each night to help your body recover from workouts and perform at its best.

Stay positive: Finally, it's important to stay positive and maintain a growth mindset throughout the challenge. Remind yourself of your goals and why you started the challenge, and celebrate your progress and accomplishments along the way.

In conclusion, preparing mentally and physically for a 30-day fitness challenge is essential for success. By building a support system, getting organized, focusing on nutrition, practicing mindfulness and relaxation techniques, getting enough sleep, and staying positive, you can ensure that you are fully prepared for the challenge ahead.

2

CHAPTER ONE

A breakdown of the daily workout routine for the 30-day fitness challenge:

Warm-up: Start each workout with a 5-10 minute warm-up to get your heart rate up and prepare your muscles for exercise. This could include light cardio exercises like jumping jacks, jumping rope, or jogging in place.

Resistance training: Resistance training is an important part of any fitness challenge, as it helps to build muscle and increase strength. This could include exercises like squats, lunges, push-ups, and weightlifting exercises. Aim to complete 3-4 sets of 8-12 repetitions for each exercise.

Cardio: Cardiovascular exercise helps to improve endurance,

burn calories, and promote overall health. This could include exercises like running, cycling, or jumping rope. Aim to complete 20-30 minutes of cardio exercise each day.

Core work: Strengthening your core can help to improve posture, balance, and overall fitness. This could include exercises like crunches, planks, and bicycle crunches. Aim to complete 3 sets of 10-15 repetitions for each exercise.

Stretching: Stretching is an important part of any workout routine, as it helps to reduce muscle soreness, improve flexibility, and prevent injury. This could include stretching exercises like yoga poses, foam rolling, or static stretching. Aim to spend 5-10 minutes stretching at the end of each workout.

Rest and recovery: Rest and recovery are essential components of any fitness challenge, as they allow your body to repair and rebuild muscle. Aim to get enough sleep each night, and take a rest day if you're feeling tired or experiencing muscle soreness.

In conclusion, a well-rounded daily workout routine for the 30-day fitness challenge should include a warm-up, resistance training, cardio, core work, stretching, and rest and recovery. By focusing on different aspects of fitness, you can ensure that you're making progress and reaching your goals.

Explanation of each exercise and its benefits:

Squats: Squats are a full-body exercise that strengthen the legs, hips, and lower back. They work the quadriceps, hamstrings, and glutes, and can also improve balance and stability. To perform a squat, stand with your feet shoulder-width apart and lower your body as if you were sitting back into a chair, keeping your weight in your heels. Push back up to the starting position, and repeat for 8-12 repetitions.

Lunges: Lunges are a great exercise for the legs, hips, and glutes, and help to improve balance and stability. To perform a lunge, step forward with one foot and lower your body until your front thigh is parallel to the ground and your back knee is just above the floor. Push back up to the starting position and repeat with the opposite leg.

Push-ups: Push-ups are a classic upper-body exercise that target the chest, shoulders, and triceps. They also work the core and lower body, and can improve upper body strength and stability. To perform a push-up, start in a plank position with your hands slightly wider than shoulder-width apart. Lower your body until your chest touches the ground, then push back up to the starting position.

Weightlifting exercises: Weightlifting exercises are a great way to build muscle and increase strength. These exercises could include bicep curls, tricep extensions, and shoulder presses, and can be performed with weights or resistance bands. To perform a weightlifting exercise, start with light weights and gradually increase the weight as you become stronger.

Running: Running is a great cardiovascular exercise that can improve endurance and overall health. To get started, aim to run for 5-10 minutes each day, and gradually increase the duration of your runs as you become more fit.

Cycling: Cycling is a low-impact exercise that is great for cardiovascular health and improving endurance. You can cycle indoors on a stationary bike, or outdoors on a road or mountain bike. Aim to cycle for 20-30 minutes each day, and gradually increase the intensity of your rides as you become more fit.

Jumping rope: Jumping rope is a high-intensity cardio exercise that is great for burning calories and improving endurance. To get started, aim to jump rope for 1-2 minutes each day, and gradually increase the duration of your jumps as you become more fit.

In conclusion, each exercise has its own unique benefits, and by incorporating a variety of exercises into your daily workout routine, you can ensure that you're targeting different muscle groups and improving your overall fitness.

Detailed explanation of how to properly perform each exercise:

Squats:
   Stand with your feet shoulder-width apart and your arms by your sides.
   Lower your body as if you were sitting back into a chair, keeping your weight in your heels.
   Push back up to the starting position, and repeat for 8-12 repetitions.

Lunges:
   Stand with your feet hip-width apart and your hands on your hips.
   Step forward with one foot and lower your body until your front thigh is parallel to the ground and your back knee is just above the floor.
   Push back up to the starting position and repeat with the opposite leg.

Push-ups:
   Start in a plank position with your hands slightly wider than shoulder-width apart and your feet together.
   Lower your body until your chest touches the ground, then push back up to the starting position.

Weightlifting exercises:
   Stand with your feet hip-width apart and a weight in each hand.
   Perform the desired exercise (e.g. bicep curl, tricep extension,

shoulder press) according to its specific instructions, making sure to keep your form proper throughout the exercise.

Running:
Begin by jogging in place to warm up for a few minutes.
Start running at a comfortable pace, and gradually increase the intensity of your runs as you become more fit.

Cycling:
Warm up by riding at a slow pace for 5-10 minutes.
Increase the intensity of your ride to a moderate pace, and gradually increase the intensity as you become more fit.

Jumping rope:
Stand with your feet hip-width apart and a jump rope in your hands.
Begin by jumping slowly, and gradually increase the intensity of your jumps as you become more fit.
It's important to keep proper form during each exercise to prevent injury and ensure that you're targeting the correct muscle groups. If you're unsure how to perform a particular exercise, consider seeking the guidance of a personal trainer or physical therapist.

Tips for maximizing results during the 30-day fitness challenge:

Hydrate: Drinking plenty of water before, during, and after each workout is essential for optimal performance and recovery.

Proper nutrition: Eating a balanced diet that includes plenty of fruits, vegetables, lean protein, and whole grains can help provide the energy and nutrients your body needs to perform at its best.

Get enough sleep: Aim for 7-9 hours of sleep each night to allow your body to recover from each workout and prepare for the next day.

Consistency is key: Make a commitment to working out every day during the challenge, and stick to it even if you don't feel like it on some days.

Warm up and cool down: Make sure to properly warm up before each workout and cool down afterwards by stretching and doing light cardio.

Track your progress: Keep a journal of your workouts, and record your progress each day. This will help you stay motivated and see the progress you're making.

Celebrate your progress: Reward yourself for reaching your goals, whether it's with a new workout outfit or a massage. Celebrating your progress will help keep you motivated and on track.

Listen to your body: If you're feeling pain or discomfort during a workout, stop and rest. If the pain persists, consult with a doctor or physical therapist.

Remember, the most important thing is to enjoy the process and make it a sustainable part of your life. A 30-day fitness challenge is a great start, but it's important to continue your fitness journey even after the challenge is over.

3

CHAPTER TWO

Nutrition for Success

A well-rounded fitness program must include both exercise and nutrition. What you eat can have a big impact on your overall fitness and health, and it is crucial to make healthy food choices to support your fitness goals.

Here are some key nutrition principles for success during the 30-day fitness challenge:

Eat a balanced diet: A balanced diet should include plenty of fruits, vegetables, lean protein, and whole grains. These foods will provide the energy and nutrients your body needs to perform at its best.

Control portion sizes: Eating smaller portions can help you

avoid overeating and keep your calorie intake in check. You can do this by using smaller plates or measuring out portion sizes.

Hydration: Staying hydrated is essential for optimal performance and recovery. Aim to drink at least 8-10 glasses of water each day, and more if you're sweating a lot during your workouts.

Avoid processed and junk food: Processed and junk foods are high in calories and low in nutrients, so it's best to avoid them as much as possible.

Pre- and post-workout meals: Eating a pre-workout meal with carbohydrates and protein can help provide energy for your workout. A post-workout meal with protein can help with muscle recovery and growth.

Avoid skipping meals: Skipping meals can lead to overeating and can cause your energy levels to plummet. Try to eat regular, well-balanced meals throughout the day.

Meal planning and preparation: Planning and preparing your meals in advance can help you make healthier choices and avoid last-minute, unhealthy options.

Remember, nutrition and exercise work hand in hand to support your fitness goals. By making healthy food choices, you can optimize your results during the 30-day fitness challenge and beyond.

Understanding the importance of nutrition in a fitness challenge

Nutrition plays a critical role in a fitness challenge and is just as important as physical activity in achieving your goals. A balanced diet provides the energy and nutrients your body needs to perform at its best and supports the growth and repair of muscle tissue.

Good nutrition can help you recover faster from workouts, reduce muscle soreness, and increase energy levels. It can also help you control your weight, improve heart health, boost your immune system, and reduce the risk of chronic diseases.

In a fitness challenge, it is essential to consume a diet that is high in protein, fiber, and healthy fats, and low in added sugars and unhealthy fats. This type of diet will not only provide you with the energy and nutrients you need to meet the demands of your workout, but it will also help you achieve a healthy body composition.

Additionally, staying hydrated is crucial for optimal performance, as water is essential for many bodily functions and helps regulate body temperature during exercise.

In summary, the importance of nutrition in a fitness challenge cannot be overstated. By following a balanced and nutritious diet, you will not only be able to achieve your fitness goals but also improve your overall health and well-being.

The recommended diet plan for the 30 days

A recommended diet plan for a 30-day fitness challenge should focus on providing the body with the necessary nutrients to fuel and support the body during the challenge. The following guidelines can help you create a healthy and balanced meal plan:

Include a source of lean protein in each meal and snack. Good protein options include chicken, fish, lean beef, tofu, beans, and nuts.

Focus on complex carbohydrates, such as whole grains, fruits, and vegetables. These provide long-lasting energy and fiber to help keep you feeling full.

Include healthy fats, such as those found in nuts, seeds, avocado, and olive oil. These help to regulate metabolism and provide essential fatty acids.

Limit your intake of added sugars, such as those found in candy, cookies, and soda. These provide empty calories and can lead to weight gain.

Stay hydrated by drinking plenty of water throughout the day. Aim for at least 8 glasses per day, and more if you are engaging in intense physical activity.

Consider the timing and size of meals and snacks. Eating smaller, more frequent meals can help to keep energy levels steady throughout the day. It is also essential to fuel up before and after physical activity.

Plan ahead and prepare meals in advance to ensure that you have healthy options available when you need them.

By following these guidelines, you will be on your way to creating a healthy and balanced meal plan that supports your fitness goals during the 30-day challenge. Remember that everyone's needs and preferences are different, so be sure to listen to your body and make adjustments as needed.

How to choose healthy food options and portion control

Choosing healthy food options and practicing portion control are important aspects of a successful fitness challenge. Here are some tips to help you make healthier food choices and control your portions:

Read nutrition labels: Before buying a food product, read the nutrition label to ensure that it aligns with your healthy eating goals. Pay attention to the serving size, calories, fat, sugar, and fiber content.

Focus on whole foods: Whole foods, such as fruits, vegetables, whole grains, and lean proteins, are nutrient-dense and provide the body with the energy and nutrients it needs to support a fitness challenge.

Limit processed foods: Processed foods are often high in added sugars, unhealthy fats, and preservatives, and can lead to weight gain.

Use portion control tools: Measuring cups, food scales, and portion control plates can help you to better understand appropriate serving sizes and control your portions.

Practice mindful eating: Pay attention to your body's hunger and fullness signals and eat slowly, savoring each bite. This can help you to feel satisfied with smaller portions.

Plan ahead: Prepare healthy meals and snacks in advance, and bring them with you when on the go, to avoid reaching for unhealthy options.

By following these tips, you can make healthier food choices and control your portions, helping you to achieve your fitness goals and maintain a healthy weight. Remember that progress takes time and consistency, so be patient and stick to your healthy habits even when faced with challenges.

Tips for staying on track with the diet plan

Staying on track with a healthy diet plan can be challenging, but there are several strategies that can help you stay motivated and achieve your goals. Here are some tips for staying on track with your diet plan:

Set achievable goals: Start by setting realistic and achievable goals, such as incorporating more fruits and vegetables into your diet, reducing your intake of added sugars, or eating smaller portions.

Keep a food diary: Writing down what you eat can help you to track your progress and identify areas for improvement.

Surround yourself with support: Seek support from friends and family members who share your healthy lifestyle goals. Consider joining a support group or hiring a registered dietitian for additional guidance and motivation.

Prepare healthy meals and snacks: Plan and prepare healthy meals and snacks in advance to ensure that you have healthy options available when you need them.

Be mindful of eating habits: Pay attention to your eating habits, such as snacking while watching TV or eating out of boredom, and find alternative ways to address these habits.

Stay hydrated: Drink plenty of water throughout the day to support your fitness goals and maintain good health.

Don't be too hard on yourself: Slip-ups happen, but it's important not to get discouraged. Just get back on track with your next meal and keep moving forward.

By following these tips, you can stay on track with your diet plan and achieve your healthy eating goals. Remember that progress takes time and consistency, so be patient and stay committed to your healthy habits.

4

CHAPTER THREE

Overcoming Challenges

During a fitness challenge, it's common to encounter obstacles and setbacks. However, by learning how to overcome these challenges, you can stay motivated and achieve your fitness goals. Here are some common challenges and tips for overcoming them:

Lack of motivation: It can be difficult to stay motivated when faced with a fitness challenge. To overcome this challenge, set achievable goals, find a workout buddy, or try a new activity to reignite your passion for fitness.

Injuries and setbacks: Injuries or other physical setbacks can occur during a fitness challenge. To overcome this challenge, it's important to listen to your body, seek medical advice if necessary, and modify your workout plan to accommodate any limitations.

Time constraints: Balancing work, family, and fitness can be challenging, especially when time is limited. To overcome this challenge, prioritize your fitness goals, and make time for physical activity by scheduling it into your day.

Boredom with workout routine: Doing the same workout routine repeatedly can become monotonous, leading to boredom and lack of motivation. To overcome this challenge, switch up your routine by trying new activities or changing the intensity of your workouts.

Lack of support: Having a support system can make a big difference when working towards a fitness goal. To overcome this challenge, seek support from friends, family members, or join a fitness community to stay motivated and on track.

By being aware of these common challenges and using these tips to overcome them, you can stay motivated and achieve your fitness goals, even when faced with obstacles. Remember that progress takes time and consistency, so be patient and stay committed to your fitness journey.

Common obstacles during a fitness challenge and how to overcome them

Common obstacles during a fitness challenge can include lack of motivation, injuries or setbacks, time constraints, boredom with the workout routine, and lack of support. Here are some tips for overcoming these challenges:

Lack of motivation: To overcome this challenge, set achievable goals, find a workout buddy, try a new activity, or reward yourself for reaching milestones. Surrounding yourself with people who share your fitness goals can also provide encouragement and motivation.

Injuries and setbacks: If you experience an injury or setback during a fitness challenge, it's important to listen to your body, seek medical advice if necessary, and modify your workout plan to accommodate any limitations. Focusing on alternative forms of exercise, such as yoga or swimming, can also help you stay active and on track.

Time constraints: To overcome time constraints, prioritize your fitness goals and make time for physical activity by scheduling it into your day. Consider shorter, more intense workouts or finding ways to incorporate physical activity into your daily routine, such as taking the stairs instead of the elevator.

Boredom with workout routine: To overcome boredom with your workout routine, try new activities or change the intensity of your workouts. Mixing up your routine can help keep you motivated and prevent burnout.

Lack of support: To overcome a lack of support, seek out a workout buddy, join a fitness community, or work with a personal trainer. Having someone to support and encourage you can make a big difference in staying on track with your fitness goals.

By overcoming these common obstacles, you can stay motivated and achieve your fitness goals. Remember to be patient and stay committed to your fitness journey, and don't be afraid to seek help and support when needed.

How to stay motivated during the challenge

Staying motivated during a fitness challenge can be a challenge in itself. However, by implementing the following strategies, you can maintain your motivation and achieve your fitness goals:

Set achievable goals: Setting specific, measurable, and achievable goals can help keep you motivated. Breaking down larger goals into smaller, more manageable ones can also make the challenge seem less overwhelming.

Find a workout buddy: Having a workout buddy can provide accountability, support, and encouragement. It's also a great way to stay motivated and make working out more enjoyable.

Track your progress: Keeping track of your progress can help you see the progress you're making and provide motivation to keep going. Consider using a fitness journal, an app, or a tracking tool to track your progress.

Reward yourself: Rewarding yourself for reaching milestones or making progress can help keep you motivated. Choose rewards that align with your goals, such as a massage or a new workout outfit.

Mix up your routine: Doing the same workout routine repeatedly can lead to boredom and lack of motivation. Mixing up your routine by trying new activities or changing the intensity of your workouts can help keep you motivated and prevent burnout.

Surround yourself with positive influences: Surrounding yourself with positive and supportive people who share your fitness goals can help keep you motivated. Joining a fitness community or working with a personal trainer can provide encouragement, support, and accountability.

Keep a positive attitude: Maintaining a positive attitude and focusing on the benefits of your fitness challenge can help keep you motivated. Remember why you started and what you hope to achieve.

By incorporating these strategies into your fitness challenge, you can stay motivated, achieve your goals, and maintain a healthy and active lifestyle.

Dealing with injuries and setbacks

Dealing with injuries and setbacks during a fitness challenge can be discouraging, but it's important to approach these challenges with patience and persistence. Here are some tips for dealing with injuries and setbacks:

Seek medical advice: If you experience an injury, it's important to seek medical advice to ensure proper treatment and healing. Your doctor can provide guidance on how to modify your workout plan to accommodate any limitations.

Listen to your body: If you experience pain or discomfort during exercise, it's important to listen to your body and stop the activity if necessary. Overworking an injury can cause further harm and delay the healing process.

Modify your workout plan: If you experience an injury or setback, it's important to modify your workout plan to accommodate any limitations. Consider alternative forms of exercise, such as yoga or swimming, to stay active and prevent further injury.

Gradually return to your fitness routine: Once you have recovered from an injury or setback, it's important to gradually return to your fitness routine to prevent re-injury. Start with low-impact activities and gradually increase the intensity and duration of your workouts.

Stay positive: Maintaining a positive attitude and focusing on the benefits of your fitness challenge can help you stay motivated and overcome setbacks. Remember why you started and what you hope to achieve.

By approaching injuries and setbacks with patience and persistence, you can overcome these challenges and achieve your fitness goals. Remember to listen to your body and seek medical advice if necessary, and stay committed to your fitness journey.

Making adjustments to the plan if necessary

Making adjustments to your fitness plan may be necessary to accommodate changes in your physical ability, schedule, or goals. Here are some tips for making adjustments to your fitness plan:

Reassess your goals: As you progress through your fitness challenge, it may be necessary to reassess your goals to ensure they are still achievable and relevant. Revisit your goals regularly and adjust them as necessary to ensure they remain realistic and aligned with your progress.

Listen to your body: Pay attention to how your body responds to different types of exercise, and make adjustments to your workout plan as necessary. For example, if you experience pain or discomfort during a certain exercise, it may be necessary to modify or eliminate that activity.

Consider your schedule: If your schedule changes, it may be necessary to make adjustments to your workout plan to accommodate your new schedule. For example, if you have less time for workouts, consider adjusting the duration or intensity of your exercises.

Don't be afraid to ask for help: If you're struggling with a particular aspect of your fitness plan, don't be afraid to ask for help. This may include seeking advice from a personal trainer, joining a support group, or consulting with a nutritionist.

Stay flexible: Life can be unpredictable, and it's important to stay flexible and adjust your fitness plan as necessary. Don't get discouraged if you need to make changes to your plan, and remember that it's better to make adjustments than to give up on your fitness journey altogether.

By making adjustments to your fitness plan as necessary, you can ensure that your plan remains relevant and achievable, and that you continue to make progress towards your fitness goals. Remember to stay flexible, listen to your body, and seek help if needed.

5

CHAPTER FOUR

Mindset and Goals

The role of mindset in fitness and how to develop a positive attitude

The role of mindset in fitness is incredibly important, as it can greatly impact an individual's success in reaching their fitness goals. A positive mindset can help individuals approach their fitness journey with confidence and determination, while a negative mindset can hinder progress and lead to feelings of frustration and disappointment.

A positive mindset in fitness can help individuals to:

Stay motivated: A positive attitude can keep individuals motivated to continue working towards their fitness goals, even when faced with challenges or setbacks.

Overcome obstacles: When individuals have a positive outlook, they are better equipped to handle obstacles and find solutions to problems that may arise during their fitness journey.

See progress: With a positive attitude, individuals are more likely to see progress and feel a sense of accomplishment, which can boost their confidence and motivation to continue.

Enjoy the journey: A positive mindset can make the fitness journey more enjoyable, as individuals approach their goals with a sense of excitement and positivity.

To develop a positive attitude towards fitness, individuals can adopt the following strategies:

Adopt a growth mindset: Focus on the process of becoming healthier and fitter, rather than solely on the end result. Embrace challenges as opportunities for growth and learning.

Surround yourself with positive influences: Surround yourself with people who support and encourage you, and avoid negative influences that may bring you down.

Celebrate progress: Recognize and celebrate small victories along the way, no matter how small they may be. This will help to keep you motivated and on track.

Practice gratitude: Take time each day to reflect on the things you are grateful for, including your health and progress towards your fitness goals.

Be kind to yourself: Remember to be kind and patient with yourself, as progress takes time and setbacks are a normal part of the journey.

By developing a positive attitude towards fitness, individuals can increase their chances of success and enjoy the journey to a healthier, fitter life.

Building new habits to support a healthy lifestyle

Building new habits to support a healthy lifestyle involves making changes that are sustainable, achievable, and consistent over time. Here are some steps individuals can take to build new habits:

Start small: Begin by making small, incremental changes that are easy to stick to, rather than making drastic, overwhelming changes.

Set specific goals: Clearly define what you want to achieve and make a plan for how you will reach your goals.

Track your progress: Keep a record of your progress and hold yourself accountable for sticking to your new habits.

Create a routine: Incorporate your new habits into a routine, such as making exercise a part of your morning or evening routine, or planning healthy meals ahead of time.

Reward yourself: Reward yourself for sticking to your new habits, such as treating yourself to a favorite activity or food after a workout.

Be persistent: Building new habits takes time and effort, but persistence is key. If you slip up, don't give up – just get back on track.

Surround yourself with supportive people: Seek out friends and family who support your goals and are willing to help you stay on track.

By following these steps, individuals can effectively build new habits that support a healthy lifestyle and help them reach their fitness goals. Keep in mind that progress takes time and that it's important to be patient and persistent in order to see lasting results.

Staying focused on the end goal

Staying focused on the end goal is crucial in achieving success in any fitness challenge. Here are some tips for staying focused:

Clearly define your goal: Start by writing down a clear and specific goal, such as "I want to lose 10 pounds in the next 30 days." This will help you stay focused on what you want to achieve.

Create a plan: Make a plan for how you will achieve your goal, including specific steps and a timeline.

Visualize success: Visualize yourself achieving your goal, and imagine how you will feel once you reach it. This can help to keep you motivated and focused.

Stay organized: Keep track of your progress and plan your workouts, meals, and other healthy habits in advance to stay on track.

Surround yourself with positive influences: Seek out friends, family, or a fitness community who will support and encourage you towards your goal.

Celebrate progress: Celebrate every small victory along the way, no matter how small. This will help keep you motivated and focused on the end goal.

Stay flexible: Be open to adjusting your plan as needed, but don't lose sight of your goal.

By staying focused on the end goal, individuals can increase their chances of success and achieve their fitness goals with greater ease and satisfaction. Remember that progress takes time and that it's important to stay motivated and committed to the journey.

Celebrating progress and setbacks

Celebrating progress and setbacks is an important part of any fitness challenge, as it helps to keep individuals motivated and on track towards their goals. Here are some ways to celebrate progress and setbacks:

Celebrate small victories: Celebrate every small victory along the way, no matter how small. This can include losing a pound, completing a difficult workout, or sticking to a healthy eating plan for a week.

Recognize and learn from setbacks: If you experience setbacks, take the time to understand what went wrong and what you can do differently next time. This can help you stay focused and motivated.

Reward yourself: Reward yourself for your hard work and progress, whether it's with a special treat or a night out with friends.

Share your progress: Share your progress with friends, family, or a fitness community to receive encouragement and support.

Keep a progress journal: Write down your progress, both positive and negative, in a journal to track your progress and help you stay focused on the end goal.

Stay positive: Stay positive, even during setbacks, and focus on what you have accomplished rather than what you still need to do.

By celebrating progress and setbacks, individuals can stay motivated, focused, and positive on their fitness journey. Keep in mind that progress takes time, and it's important to be patient and persistent in order to achieve lasting results.

6

CHAPTER FIVE

Supplementation and Rest

S upplementation and rest are important components of a successful fitness challenge. In this chapter, we will discuss:

Understanding the role of supplements in a fitness challenge

Understanding the role of supplements in a fitness challenge is important for achieving optimal results and maximizing the benefits of a healthy lifestyle. Here are some key points to consider:

Supplements can support a healthy diet: Supplements can help fill nutrient gaps in a diet, provide additional energy and support for workouts, and aid in recovery.

Consult a healthcare professional: Before starting any supplement regimen, it is important to consult with a healthcare professional to ensure the supplement is safe and appropriate for the individual. Some supplements may interact with medications or have side effects, and a healthcare professional can advise on the best options.

Not a substitute for a healthy diet: Supplements should not be used as a substitute for a healthy diet, but rather as an addition to support a well-rounded, nutrient-rich eating plan.

Choose high-quality supplements: When selecting supplements, it's important to choose high-quality, reputable brands and to carefully read labels and follow dosage instructions.

Individual needs and goals: The specific supplements recommended for optimal results will depend on the individual's needs and goals. For example, a person who is looking to build muscle may benefit from a protein supplement, while a person looking to improve overall health may benefit from a multivitamin.

By understanding the role of supplements in a fitness challenge, individuals can make informed decisions about how to support their health and achieve their goals. Remember that supplements should be used in conjunction with a healthy diet and regular exercise, not as a replacement.

Recommended supplements for optimal results

The specific recommended supplements for optimal results will depend on the individual's needs and goals, as well as any underlying health conditions. Here are some common supplements used in a fitness challenge:

Protein powders: Protein powders are a convenient way to increase protein intake, which is important for building and repairing muscle tissue. Whey and casein are the most common types of protein powders.

Vitamins and minerals: A daily multivitamin can help ensure adequate intake of essential vitamins and minerals, particularly for those following a restricted diet.

Pre- and post-workout supplements: Pre-workout supplements can provide a boost of energy and support during a workout, while post-workout supplements can aid in recovery and support muscle repair and growth.
  Creatine: Creatine is a supplement that can increase strength and muscle mass, and improve athletic performance.

BCAA (Branch Chain Amino Acids): BCAA supplements can aid in muscle repair and growth, reduce muscle soreness, and improve endurance during exercise.

Omega-3 fatty acids: Omega-3 fatty acids are important for heart health and may also support joint health and reduce inflammation.

It is important to note that not all supplements are necessary or appropriate for everyone, and it is best to consult a healthcare professional before starting any supplement regimen. Supplements should not be used as a substitute for a healthy diet, but rather as an addition to support overall health and fitness goals.

The importance of rest and recovery

Rest and recovery are crucial components of a successful fitness challenge, and are often overlooked in the pursuit of progress and results. Here are some key points to consider:

Aid in muscle repair: Rest and recovery allow the body to repair and build muscle tissue, leading to improved strength and performance.

Reduce risk of injury: Over-training or insufficient rest can lead to increased risk of injury and decreased performance. Allowing the body adequate time to recover can reduce the risk of injury and promote overall health and wellness.

Improve mental well-being: Rest and recovery can also benefit mental well-being by reducing stress and allowing the body and mind to recharge.

Balance exercise and rest: To maximize the benefits of a fitness challenge, it's important to balance intense exercise with adequate rest and recovery. This can involve taking a rest day, stretching, and foam rolling, as well as getting quality sleep.

Listen to your body: Everyone's recovery needs are different, and it's important to listen to your body and allow for sufficient rest when needed. This may involve adjusting your workout schedule or taking an additional rest day.

By prioritizing rest and recovery, individuals can support their overall health and fitness goals, and maximize the benefits of their fitness challenge. Remember, rest and recovery are just as important as exercise in promoting overall health and wellness.

Tips for getting quality sleep

Quality sleep is essential for rest and recovery, and can have a significant impact on overall health and well-being. Here are some tips for getting quality sleep:

Establish a consistent sleep schedule: Try to go to bed and wake up at the same time every day, even on weekends. This helps regulate the body's circadian rhythm and promote better sleep.

Create a sleep-conducive environment: Keep the bedroom cool, dark, and quiet, and remove electronic devices such as smartphones and televisions.

Relax before bed: Engage in relaxing activities such as reading, listening to soothing music, or taking a warm bath before bed to promote sleep.

Avoid caffeine, alcohol, and nicotine: Consuming these substances can disrupt sleep and affect the quality of sleep. It's best to avoid consuming these substances, particularly in the hours leading up to bedtime.

Exercise regularly: Regular physical activity can promote better sleep, but it's best to avoid vigorous exercise in the hours leading up to bedtime.

Limit screen time: The blue light emitted by electronic devices can disrupt sleep patterns, so it's best to limit screen time in the hours leading up to bedtime and to use blue light blocking technology.

Avoid napping during the day: While napping can be beneficial for some people, excessive napping during the day can disrupt nighttime sleep.

By implementing these tips, individuals can improve the quality of their sleep and support overall health and well-being. Remember, the quality and quantity of sleep can have a significant impact on overall health, and it's important to prioritize sleep as part of a healthy lifestyle.

7

CONCLUSION

The 30-day fitness challenge book is a comprehensive guide designed to help individuals adopt a healthy and active lifestyle. The book provides a structured 30-day plan that includes a combination of physical activity and nutrition recommendations to achieve the desired results.

Throughout the 30 days, the book encourages the reader to make gradual changes in their habits and lifestyle to develop a sustainable fitness routine. The exercises and workouts included in the book are designed to target all major muscle groups, promoting overall strength and conditioning. Additionally, the nutrition recommendations focus on promoting healthy food choices and portion control, helping to encourage weight loss and improved overall health.

One of the strengths of the book is its focus on consistency and gradual progress. Instead of promoting drastic changes, the book encourages the reader to adopt a gradual approach, making small changes each day to develop healthy habits. This approach is more sustainable and less likely to result in burnout or giving up on the fitness plan.

Furthermore, the book provides a range of exercises and work-out options, allowing the reader to choose the exercises that best suit their individual needs and fitness level. This makes the book suitable for individuals of all fitness levels, from beginners to experienced fitness enthusiasts.

In conclusion, the 30-day fitness challenge book is an excellent resource for individuals looking to adopt a healthier lifestyle. Its structured approach, focus on gradual progress, and range of exercise and nutrition options make it a comprehensive guide for anyone looking to improve their physical fitness and overall health.